LivingWise Project

LWP brings the light of wisdom and wellness to the world. With a focus on authentic knowledge, LWP aims to help people cope with the strains of modern lifestyles and live more conscious and contented lives.

For more wisdom & wellness, visit:
www.livingwiseproject.com

editorial note

This inaugural issue of the LivingWise Project is a special milestone for us. We hope this new format will allow you to engage with our quality content in yet another effective and desirable way.

LWP is not about preaching or philosophising but is only interested in helping to raise consciousness among people by spreading *sattva* (Sanskrit for 'purity') in the world.

A variety of spiritual processes find their place on LWP, from mindfulness to self-enquiry to meditation. What is culled out are tips and tricks that fall within the realm of pop spirituality.

We hope you will enjoy reading this issue and be wiser for it!

LWP

The LivingWise Project Digest
Issue No.1

Copyright © 2017

CONTENTS

Nothing can harm you as much as your own thoughts unguarded.

- Gautama Buddha

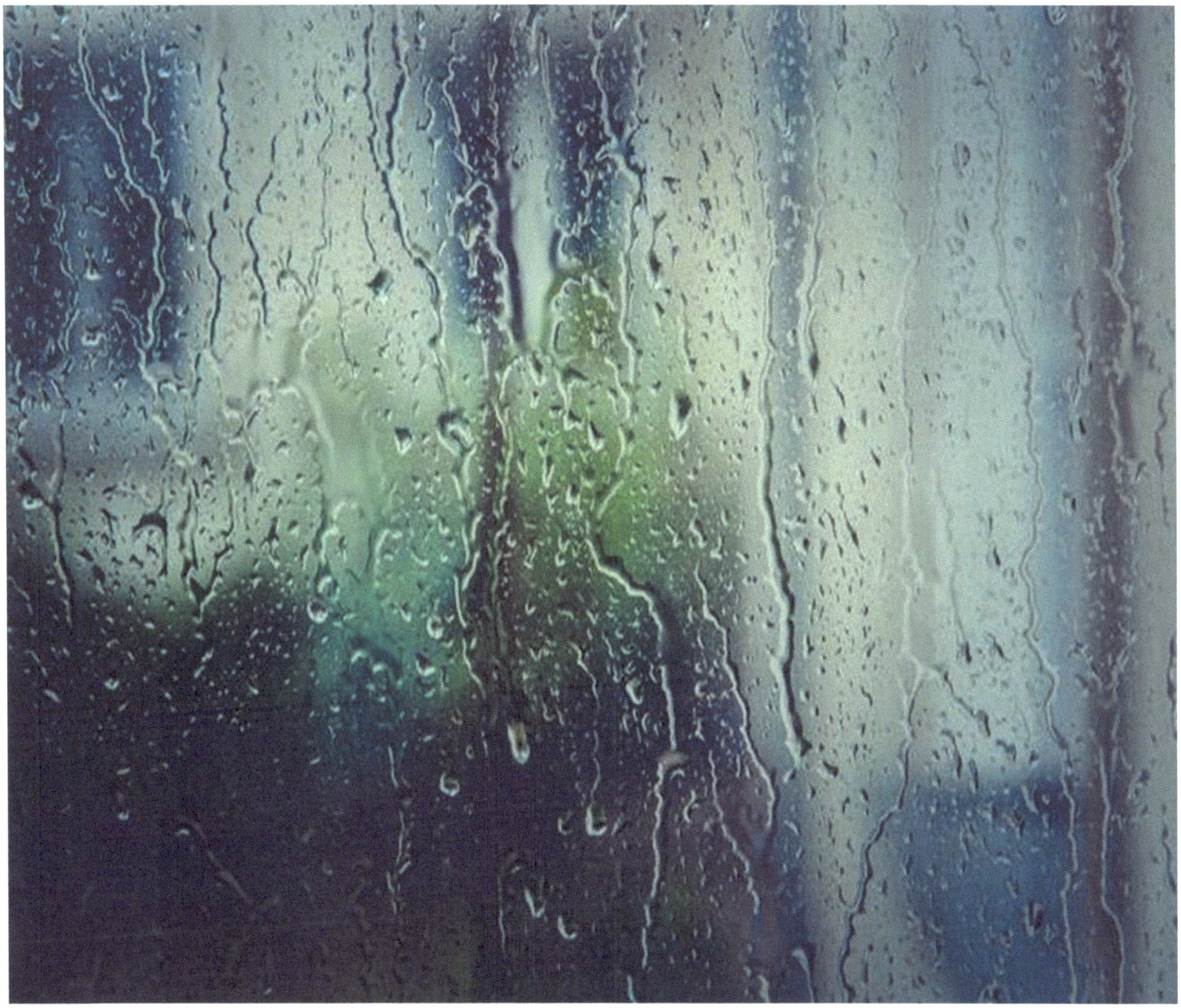

Breathe & Let It R.A.I.N.

ISABELLA CONVERTINI

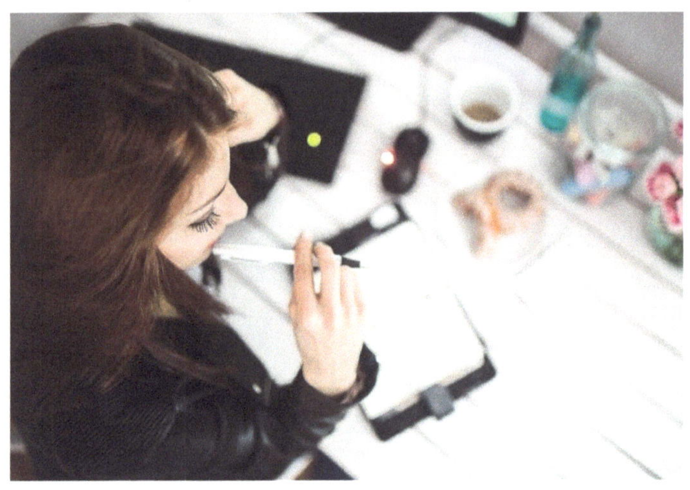

Our lives are a constant flow of emotions, which are essential to what it means to be human.

Pause for a moment and think about all the different emotions you've experienced so far today, from pleasant (e.g. joy, satisfaction, amusement, calm…), to unpleasant (e.g. anger, frustration, boredom, embarrassment…), with different degrees of intensity.

In my experience, it's quite common for people to approach mindfulness practices moved by a desire to better deal with strong, unpleasant emotions, such as anxiety, fear, grief, shame…the list goes on.

Besides the long-term benefits of practicing mindfulness in terms of self-awareness and self-regulation around emotions, mindfulness also offers some useful "tools" to deal with emotions in the moment, as they happen.

"

My favourite is called R.A.I.N., a 4-step practice that often comes to my rescue when I am overwhelmed by emotions. Here's how it works:

Recognise: This is step number one – being able to recognise that you are experiencing an emotion, and being able to name it.

It sounds simple and maybe even obvious, but believe me, for most of us it takes a while before we realise what's going on with us and it's often after we've been surprised by our own reaction to a certain situation.

As kids, we are taught how to recognise letters, numbers, colours, tastes but usually not emotions, and so as adults, the best answer we can give to a sincere "How are you feeling?" is somewhere between "good" and "OK".

The next time you recognise that an emotional state has arisen, go ahead and name it. Sometimes it could even be a cluster of emotions. For example, just a few hours ago, I came across an unpleasant work email and experienced disappointment, anger and discouragement.

*A*ccept/Allow: Once you've noticed the presence of a certain emotion, the next step is to accept it, and let it be there.

Our instinct when visited by unpleasant emotions might be to refuse, push back, ignore and numb them. If you've ever tried it, you might have noticed that at best it didn't work and probably made you feel even worse. Next time, try to give space to your emotions, practice being with them, without any judgment for how you should or should not be feeling.

Coming back to my example, I intentionally allowed myself to be angry and disappointed, I accepted to be with those very unpleasant feelings and silenced the voice inside urging me to quickly move on and pretend it hadn't happened.

*I*nvestigate: This is not an intellectual investigation, but rather a physical exploration of what emotions feel like.

While you are allowing the emotion to be there, bring some kind of curiosity to the experience and notice: where do you most feel it in your body? What physical sensations are associated with it? What thoughts come up? What actions would you be moved to take?

Since your body is much quicker at detecting emotions than your mind, this step is crucial for developing your ability to quickly identify emotions as they emerge.

In my example, I felt a tightness in my chest, a rush of heat to my face, noticed my heartbeat accelerating and my breath shortening.

*N*on-attachment: Finally, remind yourself that emotions are transient, volatile; they change, come and go like every other experience.

Notice how the quality or the intensity of your emotion might have changed in the short time of going through the first 3 steps of this practice. Notice how new emotions emerge all the time, replacing what was there just minutes before.

With this realisation, practice non-attachment: you are not your emotions. You are not "anxious", but "you are experiencing anxiety right now". Welcome both pleasant and unpleasant emotion as a natural part of your experience, bound to appear, change and disappear like clouds in the sky.

A closing remark: while most of us feel the need to practice RAIN when overwhelmed with unpleasant emotions, RAIN can also be a wonderful practice to help us appreciate and enjoy pleasant emotions, without clinging to them or trying to make them last forever.

Isabella is a career and transformation coach, mindfulness teacher and expert in business strategy. She has lived in several countries and is currently based in the US and works at Google.

"

Do you know my attitude? Books, scriptures, and things like that only point out the way to reach God. After finding the way, what more need is there of books and scriptures? Then comes the time for action.

- Ramakrishna Paramhansa

Harmony of Matter & Spirit, the Indian Way

SUBHASH KAK

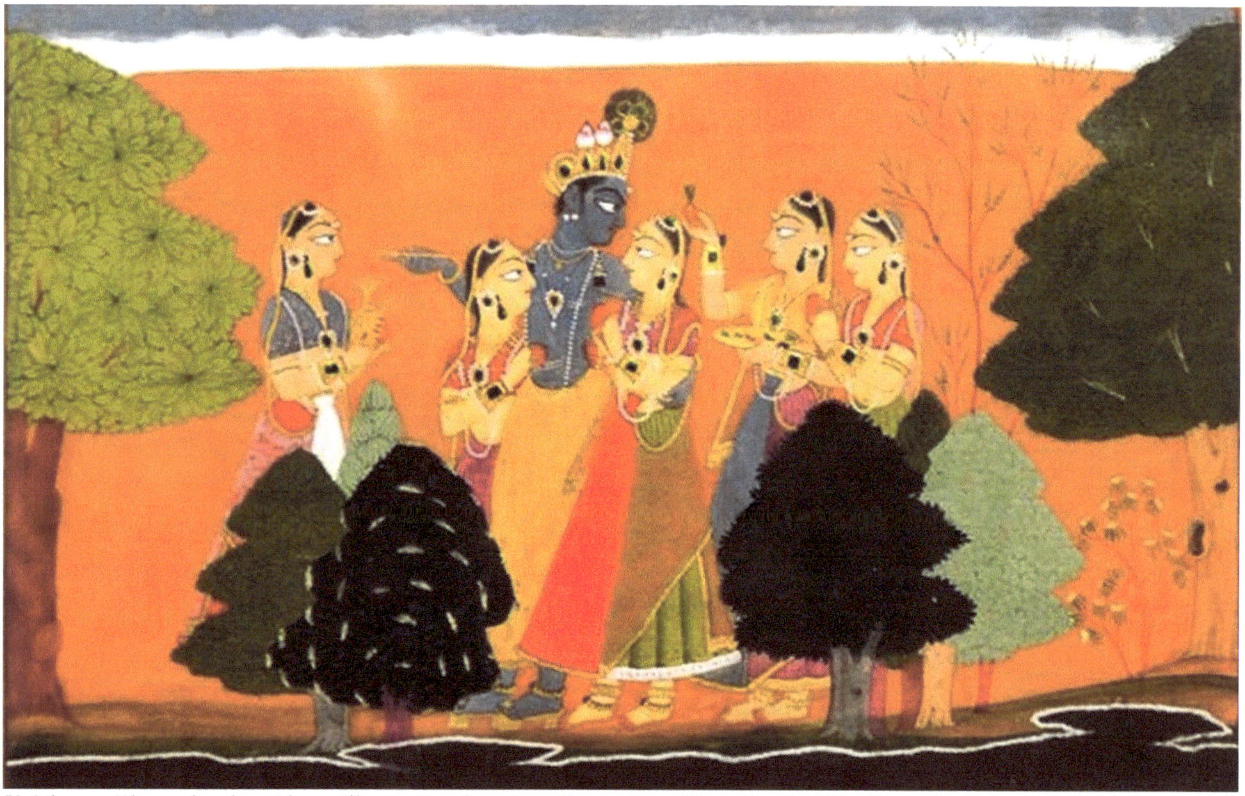

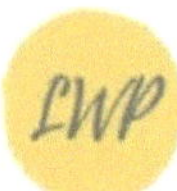

Krishna with cowherd maidens. Illustration based on the poetry of Jayadeva's Gita Govinda. Bahsoli Pahari, dated 1730 A.D.

Krishna's pranks and the love that the cowgirls (*gopis*) have for him is the frame for much of poetry, dance, and painting in India. As *avatara* of Vishnu, he is the narrator of the Vedic wisdom in the great dialogue of the Bhagavad Gita. His cowherd stories are a take-off on his other name *Gopala*, which means the protector of the world as well as cowherd, for the root *gauh* means both earth and cow.

The story of the love of the gopis is the story of each devotee for God. Krishna performs the *rasa-lila*, a dance, where mysteriously he is able to simultaneously dance with all the different *gopis*, which represents, no doubt, the mystery that the same One is able to inhabit the many.

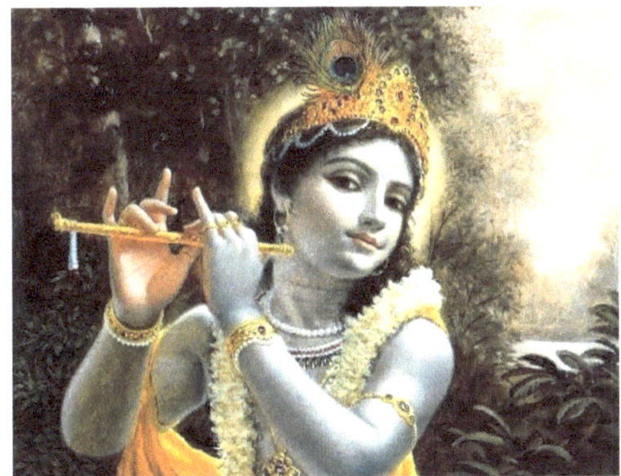

Krishna, the flute player, is the spirit that inhabits each one of us. The flute is the body, and the melody is the unfolding of our individual lives.

The love of Radha for Krishna can never be fulfilled, since the individual is forever doomed to stay apart from the Divine in ordinary experience.

In the Mahabharata, *Dhritarashtra* is the ego, *Vidura* is discriminating intelligence, the *Kauravas* are the physical desires, Krishna is the transcending atman, *Arjuna* is the empirical atman; the higher faculties are the *Pandavas*, and the lower faculties are the *Kauravas*.

"

The characters of the epics and the Puranas do not only act in the outer world; they play out our own private battles.

In the Ramayana, Sita is the intuition who has been abducted by the demon within, who must be set free by Rama, the inner sun. The demon, representing the urge to dominate and possess, has ten heads that represent the sense and action organs of the body. In the struggle between the *asuras* and the gods, Hanuman, representing the human mind that has devotion, provides critical assistance.

Although Vishnu and Shiva make their appearance generally in different situations since their centrality is in different domains, they are also visualised in a unity, as Harihara.

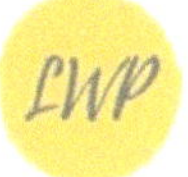

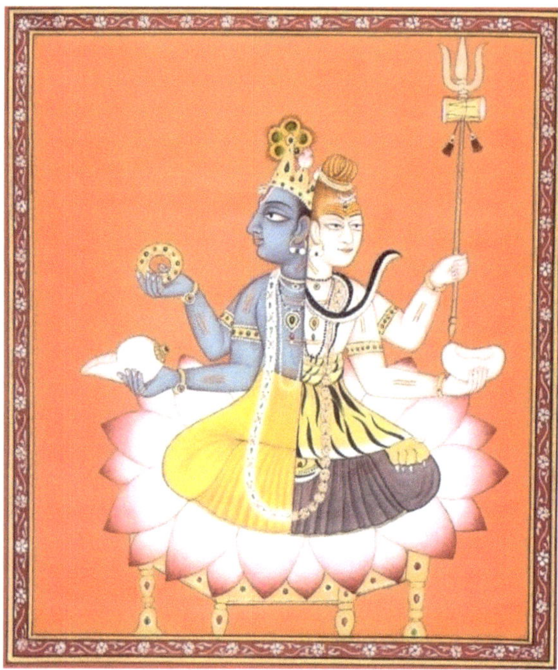

Harihara: Vishnu and Shiva as one

The Indian approach to reality is to seek a harmony that balances materiality with the spirit. It is this harmony that is the main goal of the artistic creation, and we see it expressed not only in the sacred arts, but also in music and dance.

The Indian aesthetic in an age of war

We live in an age of war fuelled by conflicting visions of reality. The mainstream cultural view is of materialism in which consciousness is an emergent process and we are primarily nothing but our bodies. Perhaps because it belittles the spirit, it is leaving many young with a sense of hopelessness. If there in nothing transcendent about life, then life may not be worth living. While some are choosing drugs or hedonism, others are rejecting rationality and joining cults. Religious leaders are stepping in with their own recipes to save the world from a soul-less hell. But their conceptions contradict each other, and although they rightly critique the materialistic paradigm for its disconnect with the spirit, they themselves remain focused on the body when they speak of everlasting life in paradise.

Because of the mechanisation of life and the expectations raised by images with which we are bombarded by the media, many are choosing not to have a family, leading to a demographic crisis in the developed world at a time when the post-industrial service economy needs more workers

and consumers, requiring vast numbers of immigrants from poorer countries. These are some of the elements leading to a clash of civilisations.

The Indian way offers a different perspective. Indian cosmology is not in conflict with science, although it does speak of the domain of spirit that lies beyond language and rational science. It makes claims regarding the nature of consciousness and transcendent states of awareness that are so extraordinary that if they should be validated by science, they would change the way we conceive of reality.

Our collective history in recent decades has tilted too much to material prosperity. The Indian way is not to reject the body, but to find a harmony between body and soul. To deal with the inevitable march of the machine and the dangers of totalitarianism of one sort or another, it provides intimations of other layers of being that lead to compassion and self-control. It opens up new vistas that shift the focus from being to becoming.

The *Puranas* have a charming story about how the gods came to become invincible, even though they started out as the weaker party. *Shukra*, the priest to the *asuras*, discovered, through science, the secret of reviving persons who had been killed in battle, and with this knowledge the *asuras* were able to subdue the gods. *Brihaspati*, who is the priest to the gods, recruited his son, *Kacha*, for obtaining this knowledge. *Kacha* presented himself to *Shukra* asking to be taken in as student. Even though he sensed danger in this, *Shukra* was helpless because one cannot turn away anyone who is seeking instruction.

Before long, *Shukra's* daughter *Devayani* fell in love with *Kacha*. The *asuras* were alarmed and they killed him on two occasions, but on his daughter's pleadings *Shukra* revived him. The third time the *asuras* not only killed him, but ground his body into powder and mixed it with the wine that they offered to *Shukra*. When *Devayani* found that *Kacha* was missing, she pleaded with her father for help and with his powers he found what had really happened.

But this time he could not just revive *Kacha* within his belly because that would cause his own death. He had to first teach him the secret of restoring life so that when revived, he would bring back the dead *Shukra* to life. This done, *Kacha* returned with the secret knowledge to the gods, who again became ascendant.

"

The coming together of spiritual India and mechanical modernity is like the coming together of Kacha and Shukra that can only be good for all mankind. With wisdom, it should be possible for people, irrespective of their cultural and social background, to live together with compassion and harmony in pursuit of a way of life that values freedom and personal creativity.

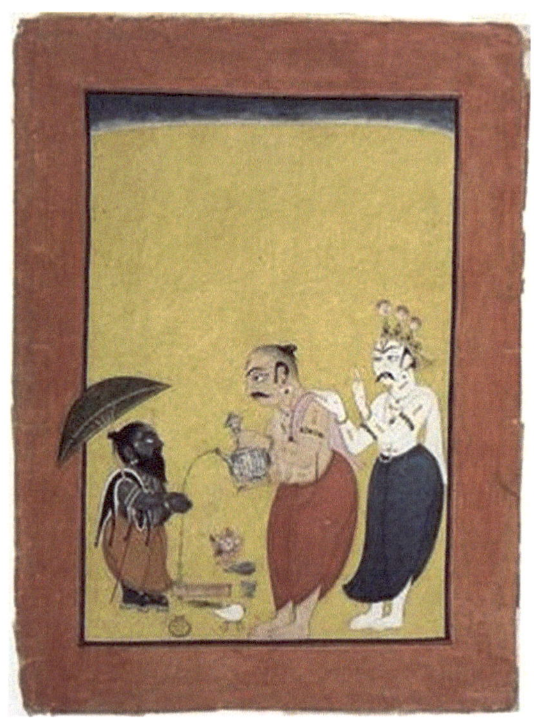

Illustration (c. 1700-25, Jammu & Kashmir, India) depicting scene from the Bhagavad Purana in which Shukra (far right) as advisor to the demon kind Bali, is warning him about the Vamana's true identity which he has recognised as Vishnu. (Source: Wikimedia)

Subhash is Regents professor at Oklahoma State University where his work has focused on artificial intelligence, quantum information, and history of science. He is also an author and Vedic scholar.

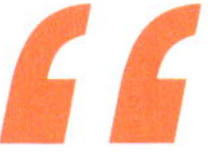

Let the world bother about its reality or falsehood. Find out about your own reality. Then all things become clear.

- Ramana Maharshi

5 *Yoga* and *Ayurveda* Hacks for Winter

LIVINGWISE PROJECT

The ancient Indian sister sciences of Yoga and Ayurveda have guided humanity to wellbeing for millennia. Both systems serve man on all three levels of body, mind and soul. At the body and mind level, yoga prescribes *asanas* (postures) and *pranayamas* (breathing techniques) while Ayurveda prescribes a dizzying array of herbal cures and supplements, massages and dietary guidelines for specific body types. In addition both Yoga and Ayurveda incorporate the science of mantras.

Being in sync with nature and using nature as a support for our wellbeing are fundamental precepts of both sciences. As winter creeps up on us, here's 5 health hacks to ensure your winter wellness.

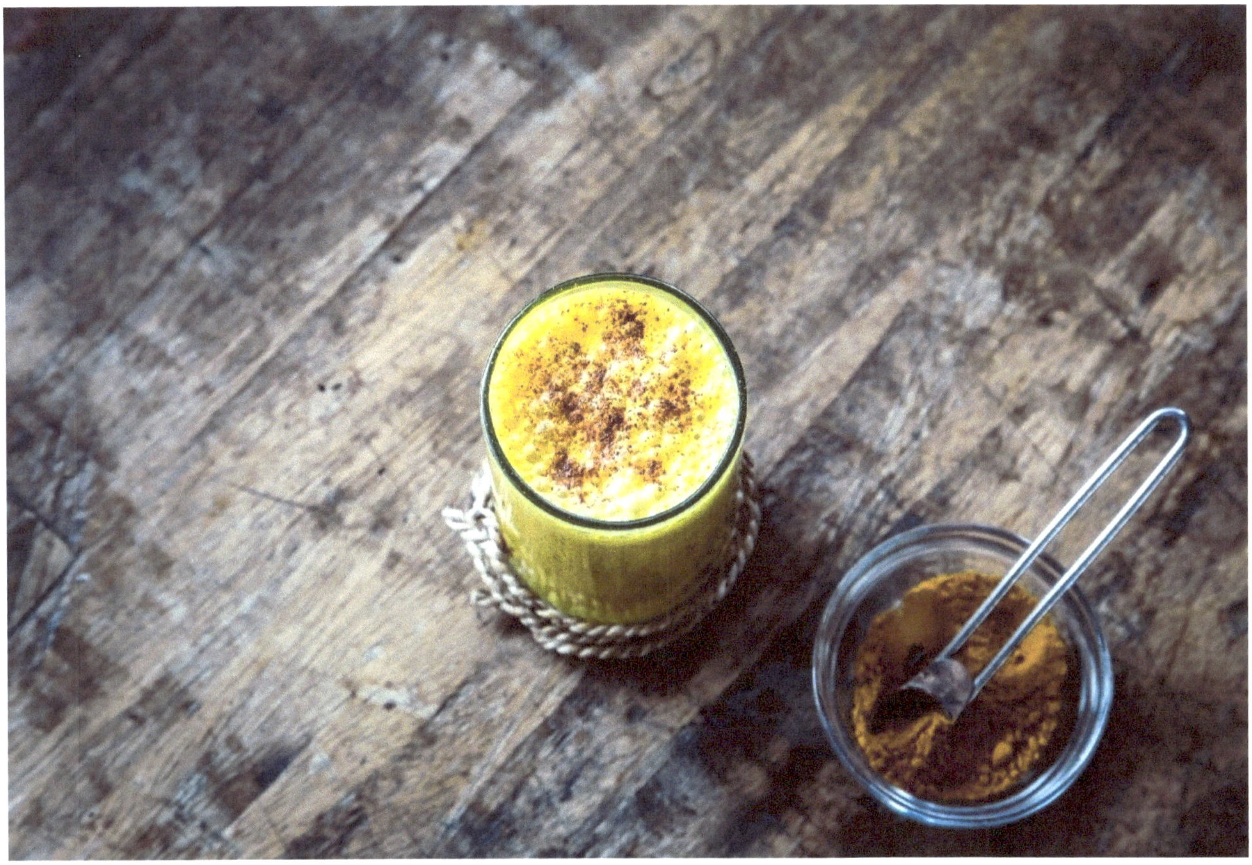

1] Golden Milk

This ancient Indian concoction for warding off the flu has taken the world by storm in recent times. If you feel even a little bit of a cold coming on, this should be your immediate fix. Simply add a 3/4th teaspoon of turmeric powder to a cup of warm milk (or tea if you want something stronger), add a tablespoon of honey and mix well.

Turmeric powder is an ingredient consumed in almost every Indian meal and its health benefits have been lauded for centuries. It is a disinfectant and natural purifier that purifies the blood, body as well as the energy system. It is also anti-phlegm, being a warm spice and remarkably, also anti-cancer. Moreover, turmeric aids yoga-asana practice, helping fight inertia and improving flexibility.

2] Ginger and honey

The winter will pass more easily if you befriend ginger and honey! Consuming a tablespoon of ginger juice mixed with honey every or every other morning strengthens immunity and is especially beneficial for a sore throat.

Ayurveda considers ginger to be one of the most beneficial spices, and it is also widely used in Chinese food and medicine. Ginger has a wide-ranging list of benefits such as aiding digestion (whets the digestive fire), soothing migraines, relieving joint-pains, killing cancerous cells, treating colds and asthma, lowering blood sugar levels, promoting cardio-vascular health and purifying the blood. Ginger tea is a warming drink that's ideal for winters.

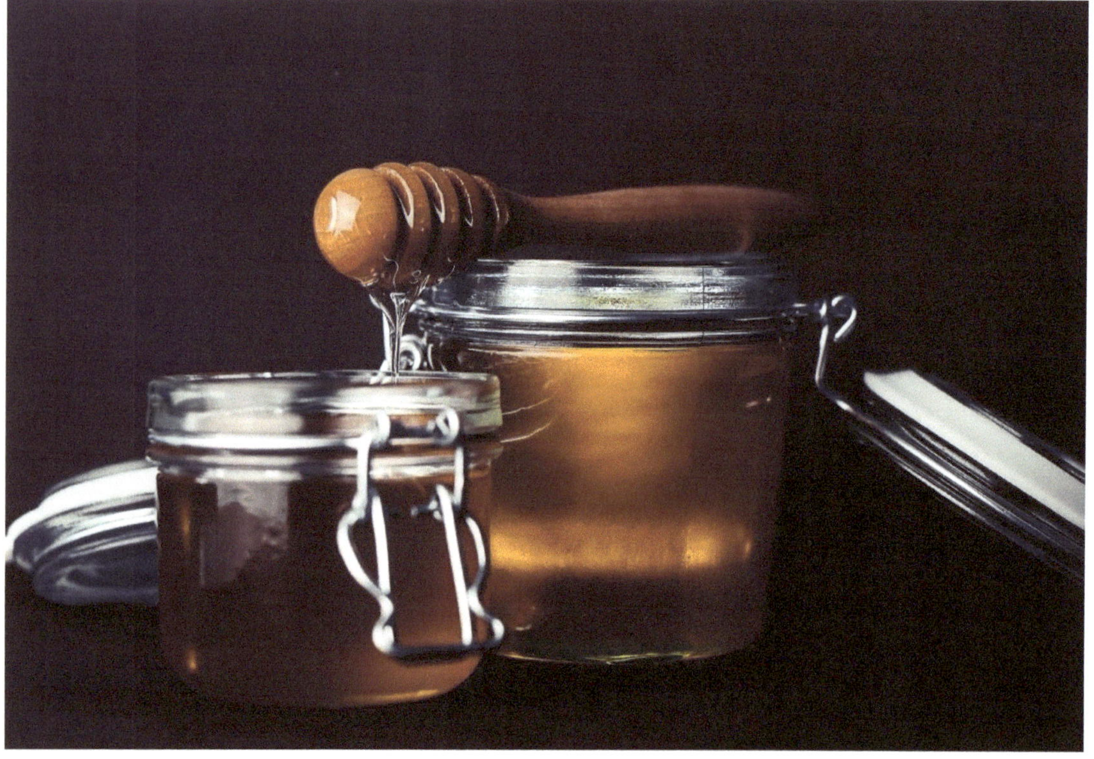

Honey is said to have a chemical composition very close to human blood and is extremely beneficial for health. It helps deal with excess mucous and asthma problems and is good for the brain, helping to keep one alert. Consuming a spoon of honey dissolved in a glass of warm water increases heat in the body.

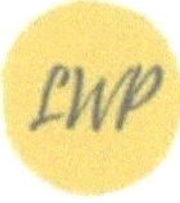

3] Yoga-*asanas*

With the external sun getting weaker, it becomes important to fire up the sun within. The Surya Namaskar or 'sun salutations' is a 12 step/pose process that was performed by yogis as the first thing they did after waking up in the morning - bow down to the sun. The sun (Surya) has been revered in Indian culture since Vedic times, for being the source of life on earth. In the system of yoga, one way of overcoming our compulsive nature (binding us to *samsara*) is by attempting to sync with the solar cycles (which are approximately 12 years long) through the practice of Surya Namaskar. Generally 12 cycles of Surya Namaskar are performed in one session followed by rest in *shavasana* (corpse pose) or yoga *nidra* (yogic sleep).

Other *asanas* that are particularly beneficial during winter are invigorating ones like the *Virbhadrasana* (warrior pose), those which improve blood circulation like the *Bhujangasana* (cobra pose) and those which improve digestion like *Trikonasana* (triangle pose) and *Sarvangasana* (shoulder stand).

4] *Pranayama*

Our body temperature is essentially maintained via the movement of air through the right (*pingala*) and left (*ida*) channels (*nadis*) of the body. The right is associated with the sun and masculine energy and therefore with heat and vigour, while the left is associated with the moon and feminine energy and therefore with coolness and calmness.

During winter, our right nostril is naturally more active than the left to help normalise the body temperature. Deliberately activating the right channel helps to effectively warm up the body. The *Surya bhedi pranayama* helps to achieve this.

Unlike the *Anulom-Vilom pranayama* technique where breath is taken in through alternate nostrils each time, in the *Surya bhedi pranayama*, inhalation is only through the right nostril and exhalation always through the left. The pranayama should be carried out gently, slowly and soundlessly.

Other *pranayama* techniques that are helpful in winter are the *Kapalbhati* (skull shining breath) and *Bhastrika* (bellows breath) pranayama.

5] Massages

In Ayurveda, winter time is characterised as a *kapha* season because of the qualities of cold, heaviness, sluggishness and slowness. At this time, therefore, it is beneficial to massage the body routinely.

Sesame (*til* in Sanskrit and Hindi) oil massages are highly recommended in Ayurveda. Sesame oil has been extolled in the ancient treatise (and one of the two foundational texts of Ayurveda), the Charka Samhita as the 'best of all oils'. It is the oil traditionally used in the daily Ayurvedic oil bath ritual/massage called *abhyangasnana*. Sesame oil is nourishing, warming, has antioxidant properties and releases impurities from the skin.

A winter ritual to follow (daily, weekly or as desired) is to massage the body with sesame oil, wait about 15 minutes for it to be soaked into the skin and then shower with warm water. Sesame oil may also be applied onto the scalp and hair once a week, to avoid dryness and restore the hair's natural lustre and balance.

The LivingWise Project brings you specially curated nuggets of timeless wisdom and freshly squeezed inspiration from modern times. For more visit: www.livingwiseproject.com.

"

Silence means you have no stuff of your own going on. All noises fundamentally began because you have created a division about 'this' and 'that'. Only when there is 'this' and 'this', there can be silence.

\- Sadhguru Jaggi Vasudev

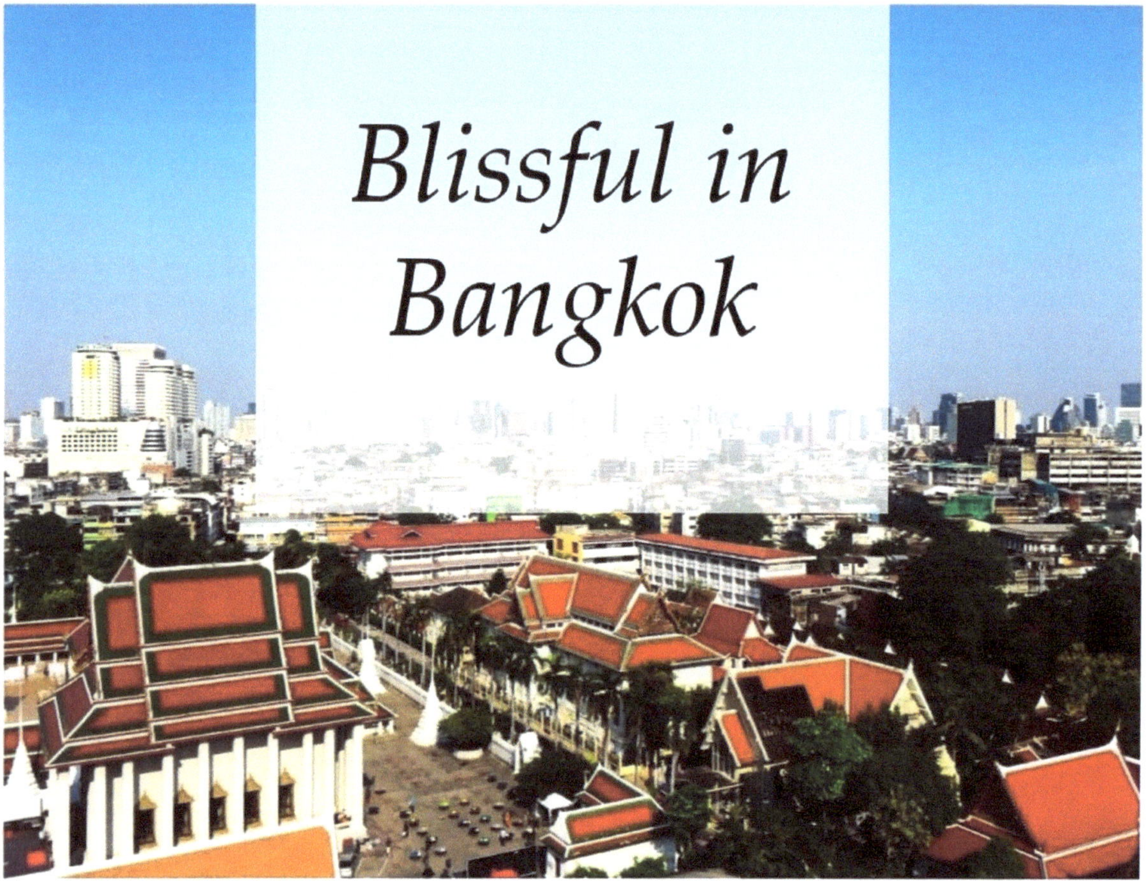

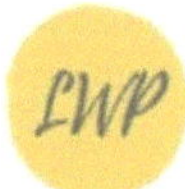

NORA VON INGERSLEBEN

Bangkok is truly a city that never sleeps. At all hours of the day and night, tuk tuks and bright pink taxis zip past street food stalls loaded with steaming pots of tom yum kung. Street sellers hawk their wares, ranging from illegal copies of blockbuster movies to counterfeit Nike sneakers. Wrinkly old women brew potions made of Chinese herbs in the city's traditional pharmacies. Bangkok is modern and traditional, Asian and Western, all at the same time. There is a buzz and energy to the city that can be matched by few other metropolises. This has made the Thai capital into not only a favourite tourist destination, but also a hub for art and design that attracts creative minds from all over the world.

"

Yet, there are also quiet spots in Bangkok where one can retreat from the city's hectic pace and let the mind wander. Right in the middle of the capital's Pom Prap Sattru Phai district, atop a hill protected by gleaming white walls, sits Wat Saket, a Buddhist temple dating back to the Ayutthaya era.

When it was first built, it was a small, rather unimportant temple. However, after King Rama I ascended the throne of the Rattanakosin kingdom in 1782 and Bangkok became the kingdom's capital, he ordered that Wat Saket be renovated, turning the temple into an important place of worship.

Several decades later, Rama I's grandson, King Rama III, attempted to build a huge *chedi* inside Wat Saket. Unfortunately, Bangkok's soft, muddy soil could not support the weight and the *chedi* collapsed during construction. Over the next few years, nature reclaimed its place and the abandoned mud and brick structure became overgrown with weeds. Slowly, it started to grow into the shape of a hill and the locals began to call it "*phu khao*" as if it had occurred naturally. Today, the 80-meter high hill, which was once the highest point in Bangkok, is known as the "Golden Mount." The construction of a small stupa on the Golden Mount began during the reign of King Rama IV.

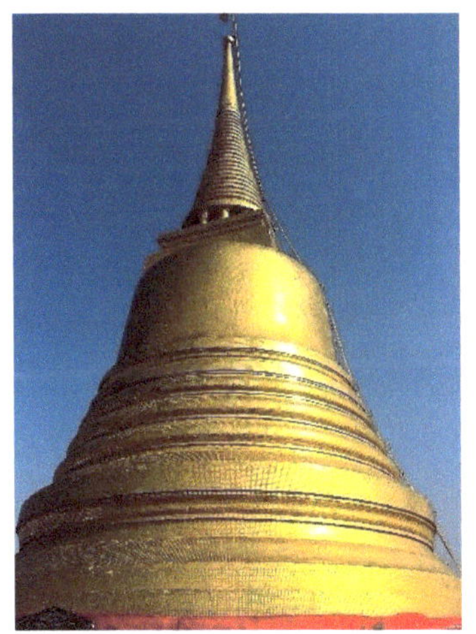

Later, King Rama V ordered construction of the huge gilded stupa that still sits on top of the hill today, glistening in the bright Thai sunshine.

Inside the stupa, one can find three statues. In the southern room, there is a 9-meter high statue of a standing Buddha, known as "Phra Attharat," which was brought from Phitsanoluk to Bangkok in 1820. In the northern room, one can find a figure known as "Luang Pho Dusit" that is sitting in the pose of submission to Mara.

Most revered by Buddhists, however, is the small shrine inside the stupa's foundation. It contains relics of the Buddha that were found at India's border with Nepal in 1897.

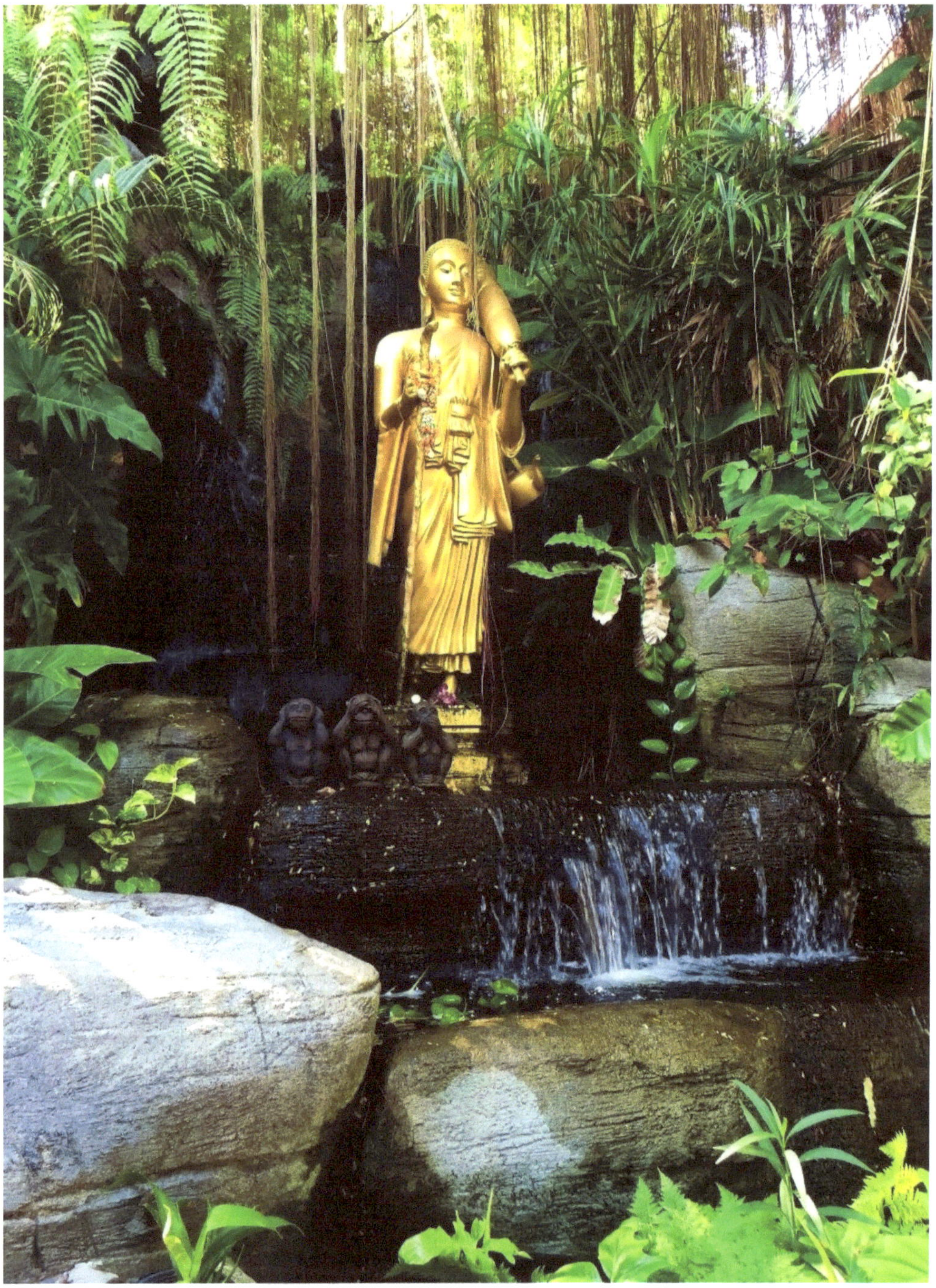

One has to climb 318 steps to get to the top of the hill, past animal figurines hidden amidst lush greenery. About halfway, one reaches a platform that is lined by a row of large metal prayer bells.

When struck, they produce a rich, deep tone that reverberates all around the temple grounds. The further one ascends above the bustling city below, the further the skyscrapers, the congested streets, and the cacophony of honking horns and screaming sirens fade into the distance. After a strenuous climb in the tropical heat, one finally reaches the *chedi*. Once inside, one starts to instantly feel calm. People from all backgrounds and ethnicities interact peacefully here, praying or simply revelling in the beauty of this special place.

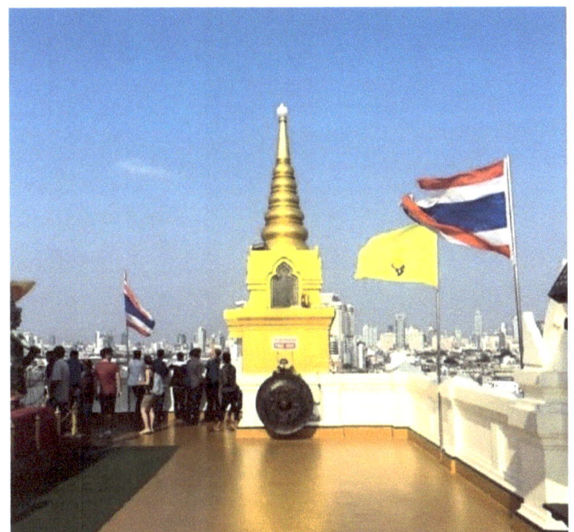
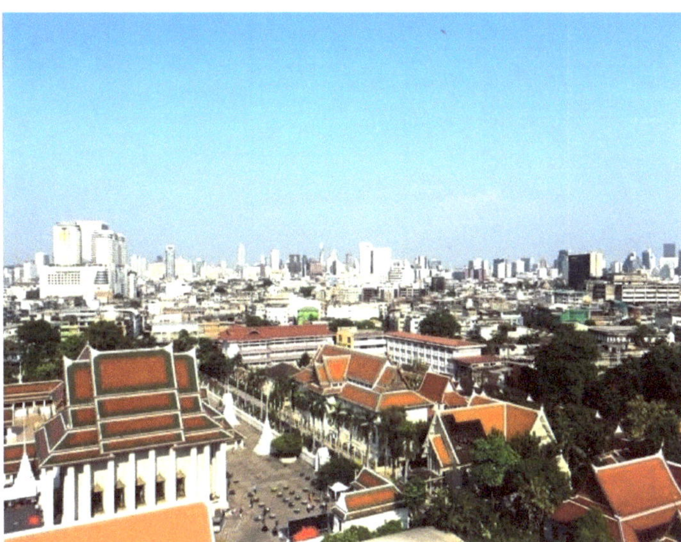

View from the top

A few steps above the *chedi's* viewing room, one can enter a roof terrace. Standing high above the city, one can enjoy stunning views of Bangkok, with the capital stretched out below like a huge quilt. It is almost completely quiet here. Only the humming sound of the engine of an airplane ascending above the City of Angels occasionally disturbs the peace. Down below, a sea of small houses with colourful tiled roofs nestles up against the tall skyscrapers that tower in the distance like an army of giants protecting the city.

In this place, one wants to become a philosopher who sits here all day, leaning against the ancient walls, and contemplates life. In any case, one does not want to leave.

Eventually, one does have to leave, though, and on the way down, one encounters an unexpected sight.

On a small platform, there are a number of statues of vultures. This is unusual, as the vulture is not an animal that is revered in Buddhism or in Thai culture.

However, the vultures played an important role in the history of 19th century Bangkok. During the reign of King Rama II (1809 – 1824), a cholera epidemic hit Thailand. About thirty thousand people died within two weeks. Many of the deceased came from poor families who could not afford a funeral or a cremation. Instead, their bodies were brought to Wat Saket, where the vultures devoured them. While this may sound grisly, the birds actually did an important public service, as they ensured that contagious remains were deposed of quickly.

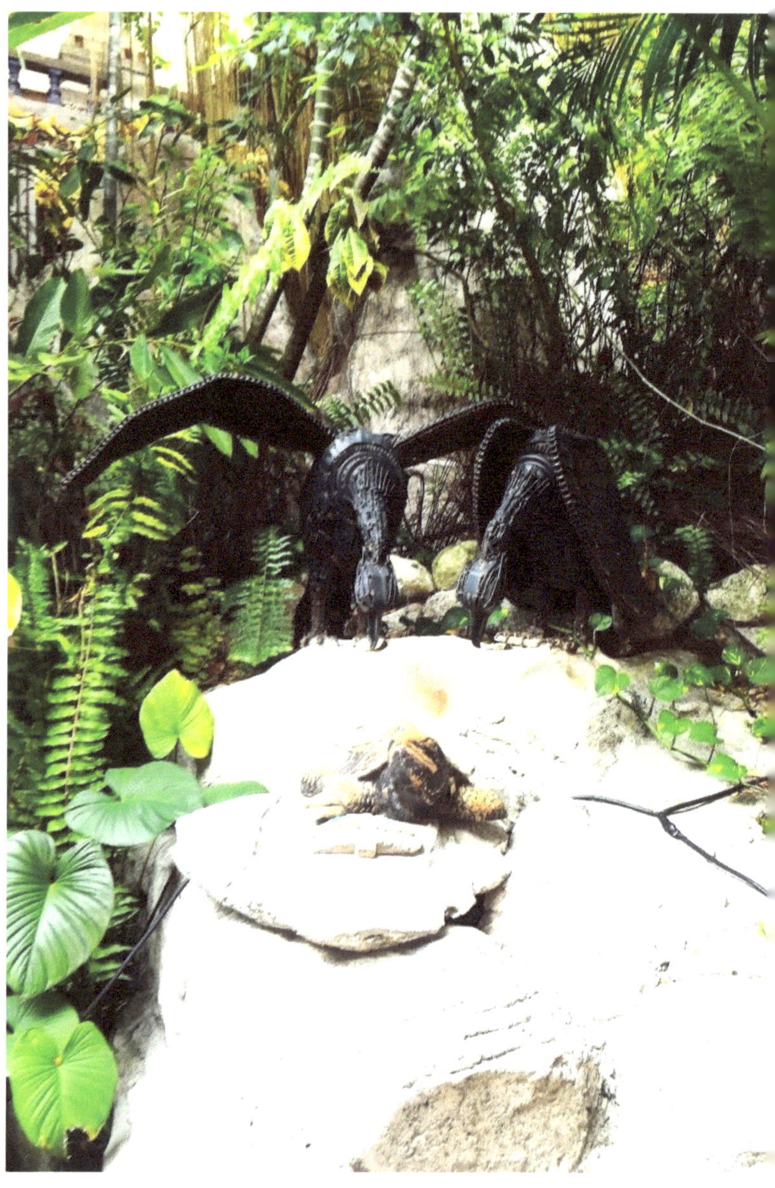

Wat Saket has provided sanctuary to many different people. The rich and the poor, Thais and foreigners, Buddhists and members of other religions all come together here. It is also a place that is deeply connected to Bangkok's history.

It reminds us of the Kings who gave the orders to build it and the workers who toiled in the burning sun to put the structures in place. It reminds us of the monks who pray here and the poor souls who died of cholera in the city's sweltering streets almost 200 years ago. Because of its deep connection to the past, it makes us think about the future as well.

Far above the city, with our smartphones turned off, we can find the peace and quiet to let our minds wander and think about the histories we want to create for ourselves and our families, the mark we want to leave on our cities and our world, and the ways in which we can provide sanctuary to those who might need it.

Nora has lived in seven countries on three continents. In 2014, she moved to Bangkok, where she has been involved in building up several tech startups. In her free time, she likes to write, travel and discuss politics.

"

Live quietly in the moment and see the beauty of all before you. The future will take care of itself.

\- Yogananda Parmahansa

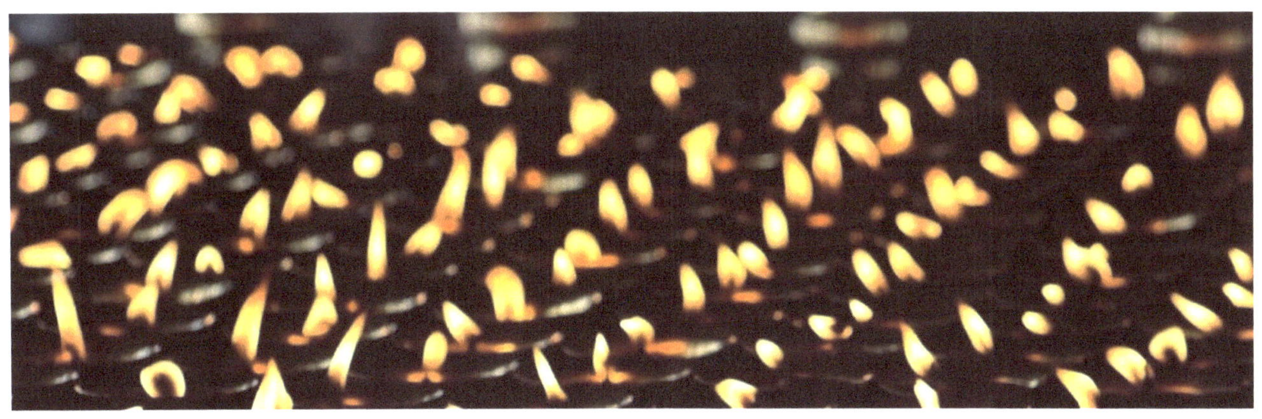

5 Days of Diwali:

From Darkness to Light

SHRUTI BAKSHI

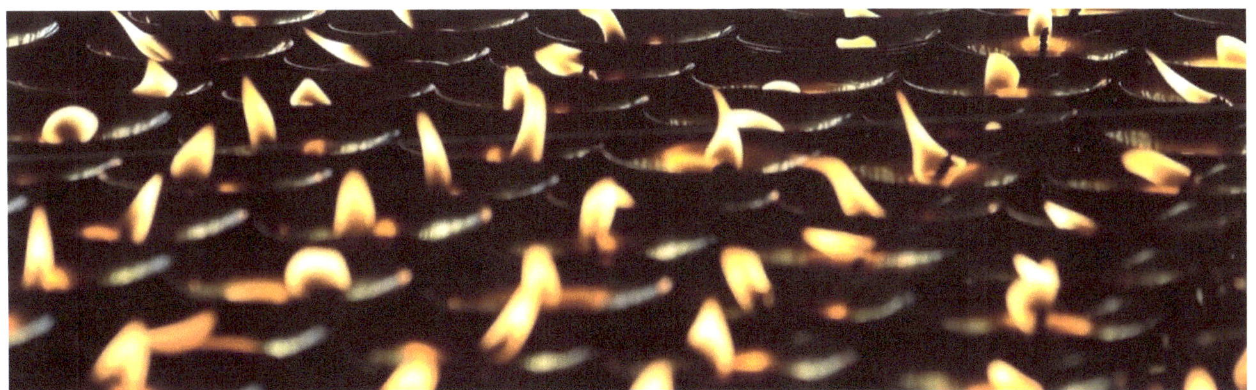

Diwali or Deepavali is the most significant and popular festival celebrated in India. "Deepavali" translates from Sanskrit as rows (*avali*) of lights (*deep*) and so this festival is the 'festival of lights'. In simple terms, Diwali is the celebration of light over darkness or good over evil, but as any serious observer knows, India's ancient spiritual traditions are not merely concerned with the simplistic divisions of good and evil. This article will attempt to shed light on the deeper context and traditions of Diwali.

The five days of Diwali

Although the main celebrations happen on the new moon day (*Amavasya*) of the month of Karthik in the Indian lunar calendar, Diwali is actually a five-day festival starting two days prior to the new moon day. The five days are Dhanteras, Dhantrayodashi or Dhanvantari Jayanti followed by Naraka Chaturdashi, then Lakshmi Puja (observed as the main day of Diwali), Govardhan Puja or Padva and finally, Bhai Dooj.

Dhanteras

In common culture, Dhanteras has come to be associated with material wealth (*dhan*) and is a day when people buy jewellery and gold and silver utensils. Goddess Lakshmi, the goddess of wealth and prosperity is propitiated. However, this day is also the birthday (*jayanti*) of Dhanvantari, the physician to the gods and the father of Ayurveda.

Dhanvantari emerged from the cosmic ocean in the mythological story of the *Samudra Manthan* bearing the pot of *amrit* or the nectar of immortality. Ayurveda is the science of inner rejuvenation using natural therapies. Dhanteras is thus an auspicious day not only for seeking material prosperity and well-being, but more intrinsically, mental and spiritual wellbeing.

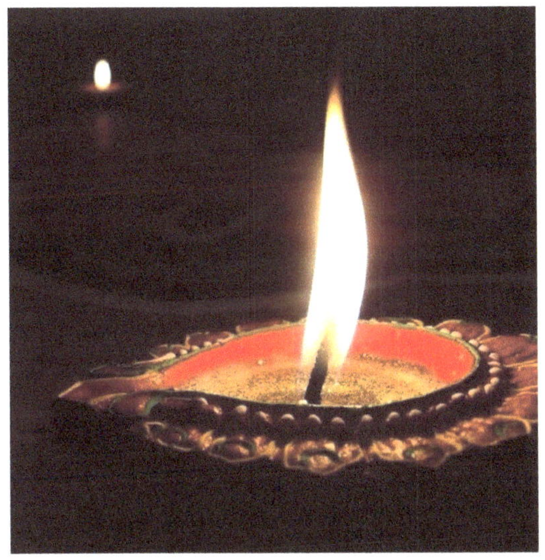

On the evening of Dhanteras, lamps are lit in and outside homes for the lord of death, Yama. This is known as *Yamadeepdaan*. This ritual represents a way of keeping away the fear of untimely death.

Digging a bit deeper into the significance of Yama, one may refer to the ancient text, the Katha Upanishad in which a little boy, Nachiketa has a discussion with Yama about the nature of life and Self. It is the fear or recognition of death or one's mortality that prompts most humans to ask questions of a spiritual nature. It is through the continual facing or probing of death or Yama that Nachiketa finds the secret of immortality.

Naraka Chaturdashi

The second day of Diwali is celebrated as the day that Lord Krishna killed the demon Narakasura. The day traditionally begins with people taking a ritual oil bath and massage or *abhyangsnan* before sunrise. The bath represents rejuvenation and outer cleansing in preparation for inner cleansing. The oil bath scrubs off all the dead cells from one's body, leaving one outwardly glowing. Scented oils are often used for their calming influence on the mind.

abhyangsnana

BODY

1. Massage sesame oil on the entire body (make sure you are dry).

2. Make a paste using the following & apply on skin:
   - 1 cup besan or gram flour
   - 1 tbsp sandalwood powder
   - 1/2 cup milk
   - 1/2 tsp turmeric powder
   - 1 tbsp milk cream (malai) (omit for oily skin)

3. Wait for the paste to dry (~10 mins) & then gently start rubbing it off.

4. Rinse with warm water. Do not use soap.

HAIR

1. Prepare reetha water by soaking reetha (soap nuts) in water overnight. The next day, boil the reetha in water (after water begins to boil, lower the heat & simmer for 10 mins). Let cool & squeeze the reetha pulp into the water. Discard skin & seeds.

2. Massage coconut oil into dry scalp & hair.

3. Pour small amounts of reetha water on the head, rubbing vigorously.

4. Wash off with warm water.

Lakshmi Puja/Diwali

The main Diwali day is one of celebration of light. According to legend, Diwali marks the day when Lord Rama returned, after fourteen years of exile, to his kingdom of Ayodhya with his wife Sita and brother Lakshman. During the exile, Sita was abducted by the demon Ravana who was later vanquished by Rama, freeing Sita. Diwali thus represents the triumph of Rama and the celebration of his homecoming. Being a moonless night, the people of Ayodhya lit oil lamps to light the way for Rama, Sita and Lakshman. Thus the festival of lights was born.

Diwali is also the most important day for propitiating the Goddess Lakshmi who is believed to bestow blessings around the earth on this day. People light oil lamps all over their houses and neighbourhoods and engage in *sadhana* (spiritual practices) to light up from within.

Govardhan Puja/Padva

This day goes back in legend as the day that Lord Krishna lifted the Govardhan mountain to shelter the people of Vrindavan from torrential rains. The story goes that the people of Vrindavan had a tradition of propitiating Indra, the god of rain and thunder during the autumn season. Krishna did not approve of this and wanted to show the people that they didn't have to pay homage to lesser gods but only to that one Supreme Being that he himself was the clear evidence of, as an *avatar* (incarnation). He started a tradition where the villagers would make offerings to the Mount Govardhan which he would accept, taking the form of the mountain.

Indra was displeased at this and struck the village with heavy rains. Krishna simply lifted Mount Govardhan on his little finger and sheltered the entire village. After seven days of downpour, Indra finally gave up.

It is this aspect of Krishna as providing refuge to his devotees that is invoked on the day of Govardhan Puja, celebrated mainly in northern India. In some parts of northern and western India, this day is considered to mark a new year.

Bhai Dooj

Also referred to as Bhai Tika or Bhai Beej, this day celebrates the brother-sister relationship. According to legend, after slaying the demon Narakasura, Krishna visited his sister Subhadra who warmly welcomed him with sweets and flowers. Even today, this day is celebrated in India between brothers and sisters with an exchange of gifts, flowers and sweets.

Spiritual significance of Diwali

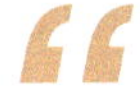

At a superficial level, Diwali is seen as the triumph of good over evil. But the spiritual significance is the triumph of the light of knowledge over the darkness of ignorance. Light represents clarity; being able to see things the way they are, free of illusion.

At a relative level, Rama represents the individual soul. Emancipating his higher intellect or *buddhi* (Sita) from the clutches of ignorance (Ravana) with the help of the power of devotion or *sadhana* (Hanuman) and power of will (Lakshman), the individual soul (Rama) emerges victorious.

Rama also represents the inner sun. In his human form too, Rama belonged to the *Suryavanshi* clan, the solar dynasty. The period of Diwali is thus associated with the sun and yogic practices like the *surya namaskar* (sun salutation) are considered important at this time.

The light we celebrate at Diwali is the light of the Self. The Self is described in several ancient Indian texts as the "shining One". The ancient invocations and mantras repeatedly invoked the light of the highest realisation:

Tamaso Maa Jyotir-Gamaya
Lead us from darkness to light

- In the Brihadaranyaka Upanishad

Tat Savitur Varenyam

That Supreme Being that is the radiating source of life, shining like the sun, is most desirable

- In the Gayatri Mantra

Murdha jyotishi siddha darshanam

Once you recognize the (Divine) light within you, you will attain perfection. Many *siddhis* (extraordinary abilities) will be awakened and your intellect will be refined and illumined.

- In Patanjali's Yoga Sutras

Amasvasya or new moon nights are anyway generally considered beneficial for spiritual practices aimed at liberation because on this day, life slows down on the planet and one is more clearly able

to realise a distance between our bodies and our true selves. Symbolically, the moon, representing the mind, cannot be seen, allowing one to more easily recognise what is beyond the mind.

The true significance of Diwali is that when the veil of ignorance is lifted, light floods in. It is the recognition of the pure joy and bliss of the Self, the celebration of life. The light is always here and only *appears* to be covered up by darkness. Diwali is a reminder of that light that we are.

If there is light outside the window and darkness in the room, the light fills the whole room but if there is darkness outside the window and light in the room, the darkness does not engulf the room. – Mooji

Special references:
1) artofliving.org
2) ishafoundation.org

Shruti is an author and the founder of the LivingWise Project. She has worked for several years in financial services in London and Paris and currently resides in India

"

Whenever I am giving a lecture on quantum physics, I feel I am speaking on Vedanta.

- Hans-Peter Durr

Remembering Annapurna

BELOO MEHRA

LWP

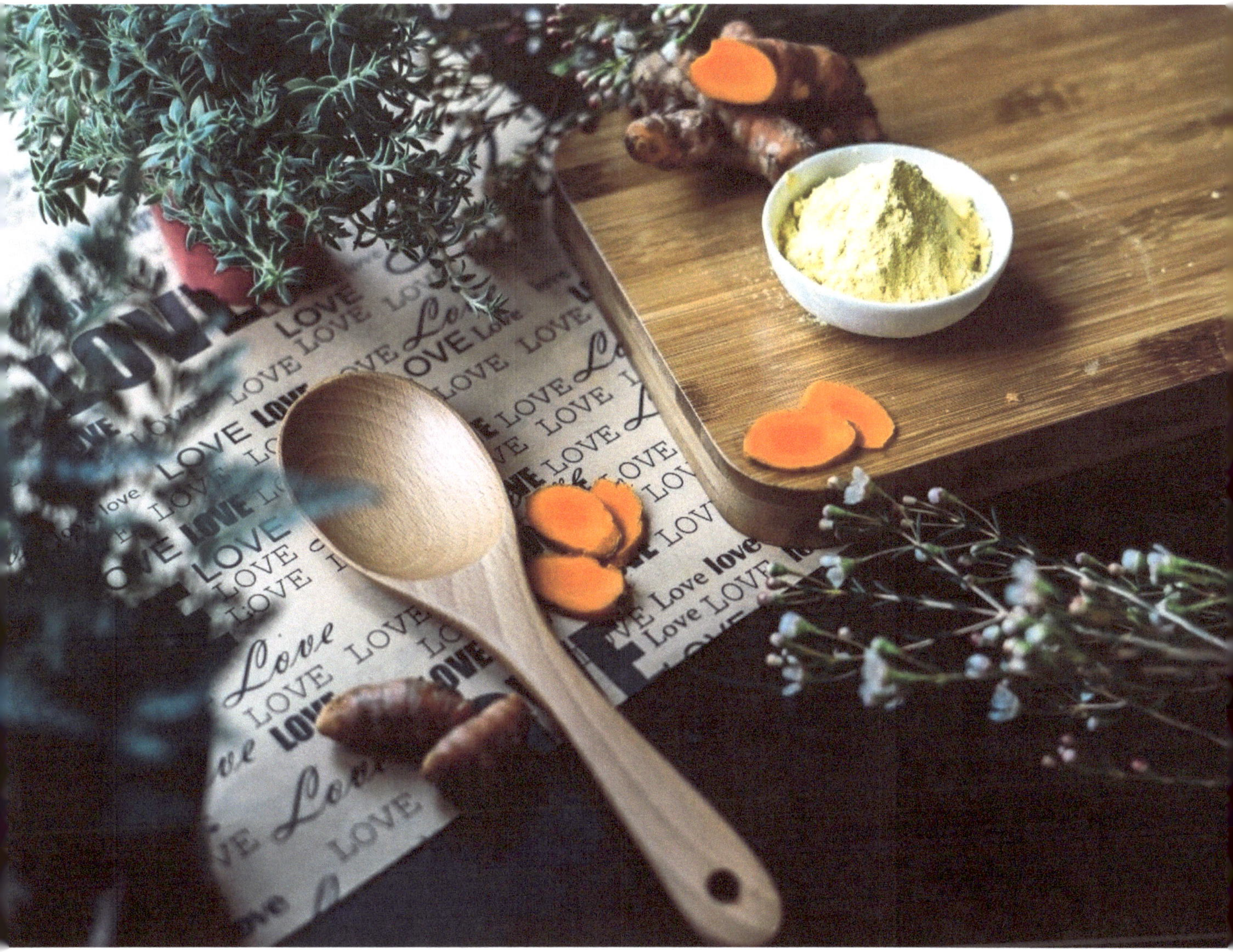

She would recite, in a very soothing low voice, almost inaudible to others but her, one of her *bhajans* whenever she was cooking. Or she would be doing her regular *japa* as she worked in her simple kitchen in her modest home in the big city. Her food tasted heavenly, perhaps because of that.

Everyone who ate even once in her home felt that 'special' taste in her food. It was not only their physical hunger that felt satisfied. Something else was being fed too. The real thing within, perhaps.

She wasn't into cooking anything gourmet or grand. There were no special recipes that she used. She didn't use any special spices or ingredients. On the contrary, the food she cooked was very simple, and simply prepared. It was basic, vegetarian, Punjabi food for the most part, and that too without any hot spices.

She never hired any outside help for any task related to cooking, even when her children were small and needed a lot of attention and looking after. She managed everything herself, in addition to her work as a school teacher which she took very seriously. Her husband had some health issues and also needed much care and special attention. She would often need to cook special meals for him. Her lips moving silently in a prayer, she would manage it all by herself.

The house was also frequently filled with extended family members and relatives visiting from other towns. They would often stay for a few days. Or more. She smilingly fed them, made them as comfortable in her modest home as she could, and even packed lunches or home-cooked snacks for them when they went outside for sight-seeing or some other work.

When her children grew up, they helped her whenever they could and to whatever extent they could. Sometimes her children would get upset and ask her why she had to do all that cooking for the guests. Why couldn't they just stay in a hotel? And she would simply smile and say — that is not how it is done. You don't bother, go and study, I will manage.

As she grew older she began to realize she needed some help in the kitchen, especially when her health started giving her problems. Though by this time the children had moved out of the parental home and the frequency of visiting guests had also reduced, she found herself getting tired frequently. She hired someone to help her with some basic food prep tasks, like chopping of vegetables or kneading the dough or some such thing. The actual preparation of dishes was always done by her. In that same prayerful mood.

Until the very last year of her life. Her failing health would simply not permit her to stand for more than five minutes without any support. And she was compelled to hire someone to cook for herself and her husband.

The children had always visited their parental home, as frequently as grown children do in a close-knit family. Those who lived in other towns would come and even stay with the parents for several days. But when her health started to deteriorate further and the diagnosis revealed a terminal illness, the children would take turns and come to live with her and their father for extended periods of time.

The kitchen was again bursting with activity as children and grand-children frequently visited. But she wasn't in the kitchen. She was however still very concerned with what was being cooked, and would give detailed instructions, in her frail voice, to the cook regarding how to prepare this dish or that dish. In just a couple of months, despite her failing health she had actually trained the cook to prepare almost everything as per her style.

And as the cook would get busy in the kitchen, sitting in the chair in her bedroom she would close her eyes and recite one of her *bhajans* or do her *japa*.

The food tasted the same. Almost. And satisfied both the physical and the other real hunger within.

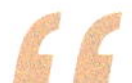

Where was the magic? In her hands? In her love for the family? In her prayers? Or all?

Now that she is gone, the same cook still works in the same kitchen of her home. Cooking for one, her husband. Or for more when the children visit.

But there is nobody reciting the prayers, silently, while the cooking is being done.

Or maybe there is. Far, far away. Or very near. Right here. Within.

Within the hearts of her children, her husband, all those who will visit her home and partake of something cooked in her kitchen, where she and her prayers are present. Always.

In all her acts a strange divinity shone:

Into a simplest movement she could bring

A oneness with earth's glowing robe of light,

A lifting up of common acts by love.

~ *Sri Aurobindo, Savitri, Book VII, Canto I*

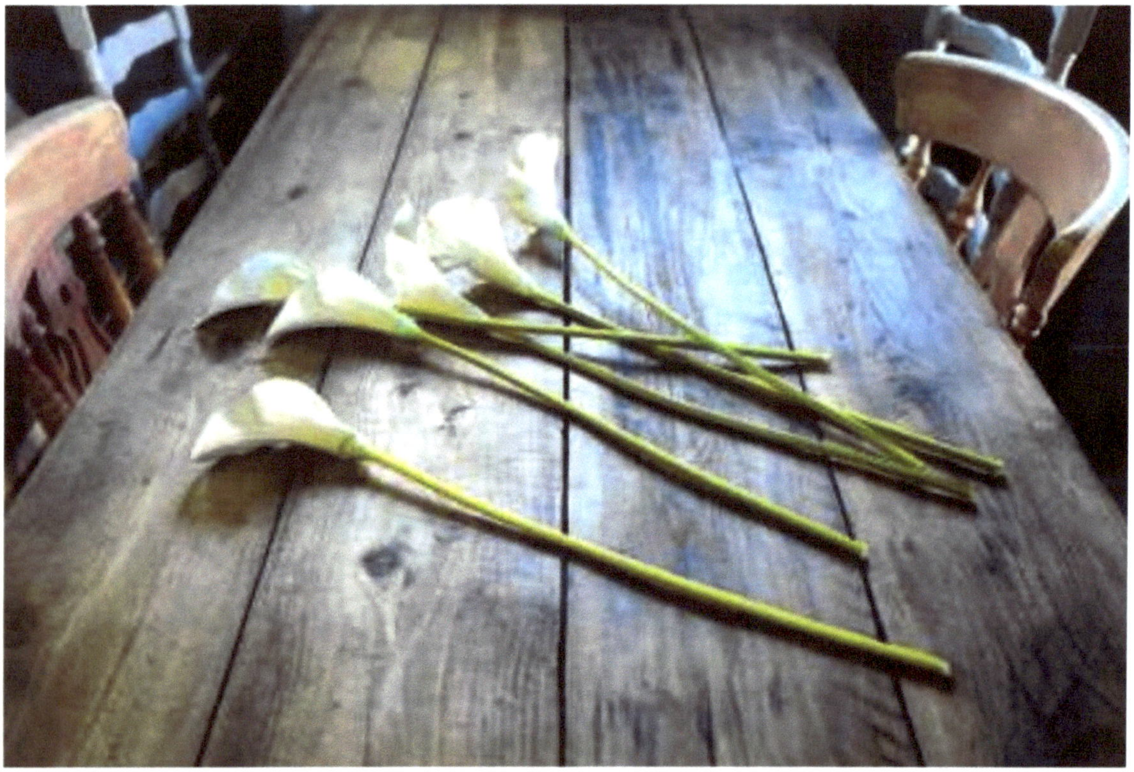

Beloo has been a school teacher, university professor and researcher. She is also an author and lives in Pondicherry, where she devotes most of her time to studying the works of the Mother and Sri Aurobindo.

"

Jnanadhisthanam matrka:

Go to the root of knowledge - Silence.

- Shiva Sutras

"Om" In Paris: Learning Yoga with the French

SHRUTI BAKSHI

When I moved to France, I packed with my luggage, a full openness to imbibe what I could of the high fashion, famed gastronomy and the much touted cultural sophistication of the country.

Stepping off the airplane in Paris, my head was full of dreamy images of the back lanes in which Edith Piaf probably once sang and waltzed around, the broody cafes in which Hemmingway once slouched over his notebook late into the night and the dazzling abodes of Louis Vuitton and Channel, frequented by the most elusive celebrities. So it was indeed completely unexpected that the most valuable import I returned to India with after my four-year Parisian stay, was yoga.

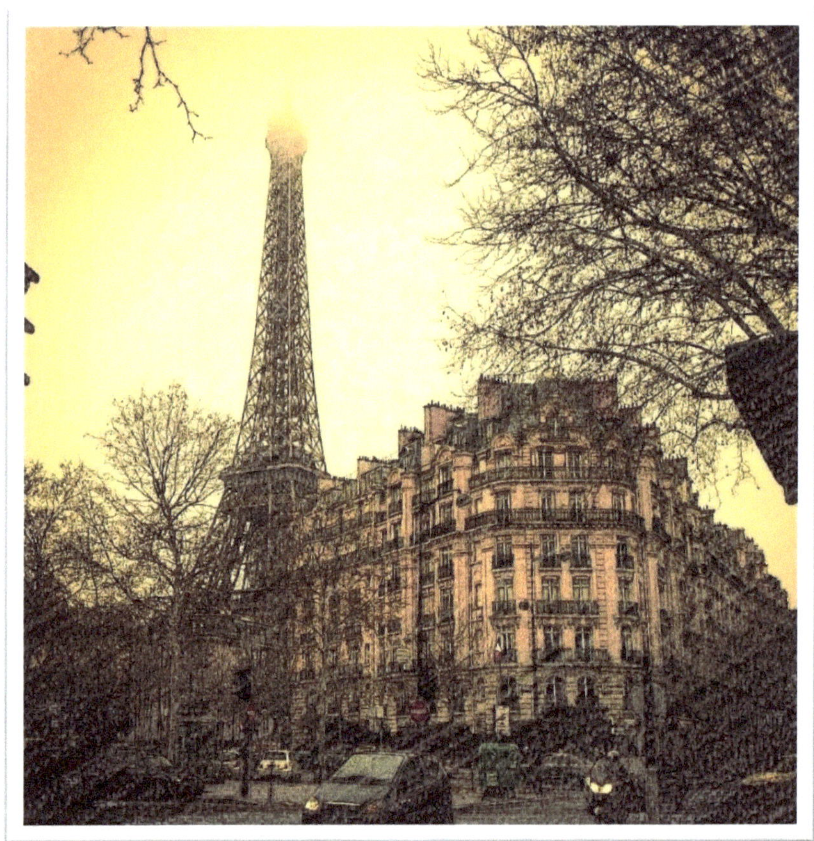

Yoga as a spiritual practice was developed in India many millennia ago. In yogic lore, the first yoga *guru,* who imparted the tools of yoga to humanity, was *AdiYogi*, or Shiva, the first yogi. Despite having grown up in India, however, I somehow managed to remain quite untouched by the influence of its more profound spiritual traditions. Perhaps it was because of the Western education I received growing up in cosmopolitan Mumbai, where Shakespeare and ballet were favoured over Patanjali and yoga-*asanas*.

My first serious tryst with yoga, consequently, was on the shady lawns of the Champs des Mars, in the shadows of the Eiffel tower. As I discovered early on, yoga classes in Paris were not only popular for their health benefits, but also great for socialising and exploring the city. Expats in Paris are inundated with choices of low priced classes in various parks across the city allowing them to gloat to friends back home about how they achieved a perfect headstand at the Esplanade des Invalides, gaining a unique upside-down view of Napoleon's tomb.

And so it was that being first generation Indian myself, I began to learn 'third' generation yoga in Paris — i.e. yoga gone from India to America and then to Europe. You see, the first globally mobile modern Indian spiritual teachers taught yoga first to the Americans, noting of course the amazing power of America to inspire, if it so wanted, the whole world to wear torn blue trousers made from thick, coarse cloth and to drink black carbonated water while feeling really chuffed about it. Sure enough, no sooner did they spot New Yorkers running to the gym with yoga mats slung over their shoulders, that Parisians and Berliners sprung into *asanas* themselves.

As I graduated from the introductory 'yoga in the park' classes to a chic yoga studio on Boulevard de la Madeleine, I learned that Parisians take their yoga seriously. And fashionably. Doing yoga is a sort of fashion statement especially among those cosmopolitan enough to have witnessed first-hand, the yoga craze in California.

While I admittedly chuckled to myself on first hearing Sanskrit chants in a French accent, my amusement was marred by my slight embarrassment at listening to 20 French people confidently chant ancient Indian *shlokas* that I did not know. What was also surprising to me was that Hindu devotional songs were played at the end of the yoga class as everyone lay prostrate in *shavasana,* soaking in the chanting for Krishna or Ganesha. As I listened, I silently rued how in India, on the

contrary, the urban elite I knew would be embarrassed to publicly engage in the same, thinking it to be regressive. Back home, the embarrassment over our own traditions was real, however absurd, while Parisians prided themselves on their knowledge of ancient Sanskrit mantras!

This spiritual enthusiasm for yoga outside India has been so great that there now exist new styles of yoga invented in the West. When I asked

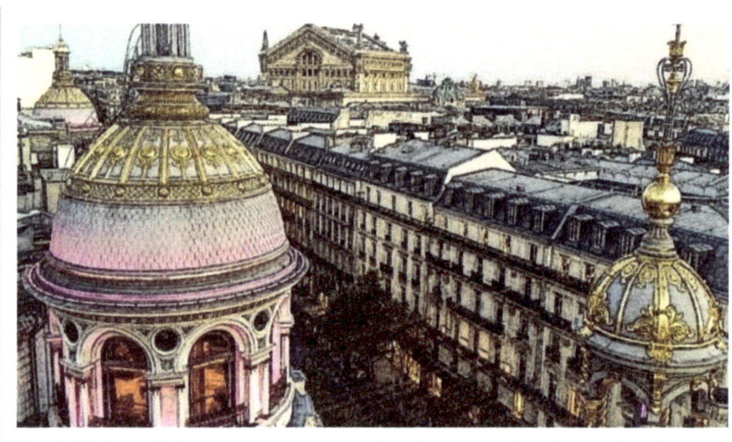

my Jivamukti class teacher in Paris where she studied the yoga form, I was hoping she would point me to some good school or teachers in India but her answer was — New York. At times though, this spiritual enthusiasm does get a bit carried away. As I matured in my yoga practice and delved more deeply into the philosophical and spiritual aspects, the yoga classes on Boulevard de la Madeleine suddenly appeared quite superficial. Some of the teachers' enthusiasm in pushing us into *asanas* at a frantic pace made the practice feel more like a gymnastics or gym class as opposed to a spiritual practice. I slowly became convinced that if I wanted to know the real thing, I would have to come back to India.

I am grateful to Paris though, for introducing to me, amid the Nutella *crepes* and *chèvre chaud*, my own Indian spiritual tradition of yoga. One feature of the globalised world is the ability of ancient traditions to carry on foreign soils. And yoga may well be the one truly global philosophy/practice, serving to bind the world together not along potentially divisive ideological, political, economic or religious, but along basic existential lines.

So in the end, it doesn't really bother me to learn it first as '*chien tête en bas*' or 'downward facing dog'; after all, an *asana* by any other name…

Shruti is an author and founder of the LivingWise Project. She has worked for several years in financial services in London and Paris and currently resides in India.

"

When the mind desires or grieves things, accepts or rejects things,

is pleased or displeased by things--

this is bondage.

When the mind does not desire or grieve,

accept or reject,

become pleased or displeased, liberation is at hand.

If the mind is attached to any experience,

this is bondage.

When the mind is detached from all experience, this is liberation.

- Ashtavakra Gita

At the Isha Yoga Centre:

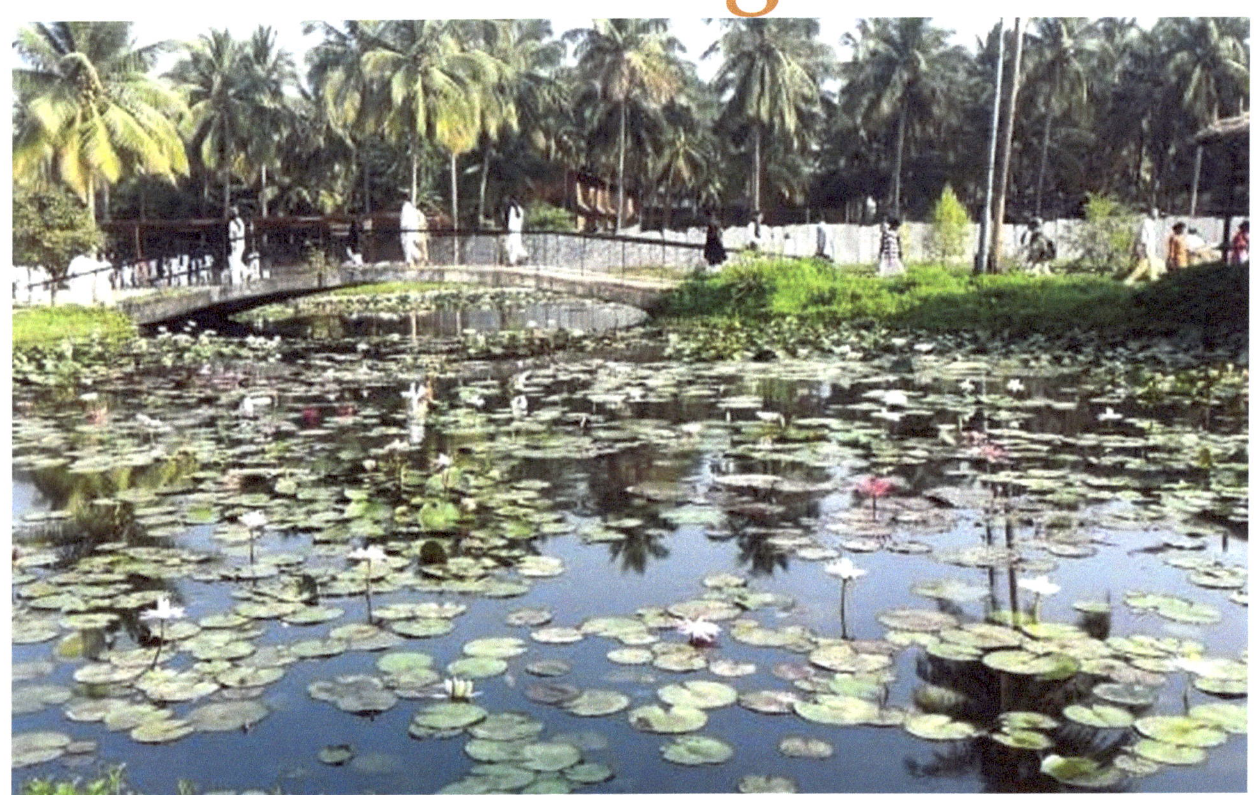

A Spiritual Travelogue

RAHUL SHARMA

Spirituality, for most beginners, commences with the excitement of wanting to know the unknown. However, this mystic infatuation lasts for a few days until one switches attention to something new and more exciting when the meditation just doesn't seem to work despite one's best efforts. Hence one very conveniently concludes, *"Life is anyway short, just go with the flow and enjoy your pizza, mate!"* I, and the people around me also probably thought that I would go down the same route. But I was wrong!

Here I was at Sadhguru Jaggi Vasudev's ashram, after a year of lengthy discussions, some deep digging into books/media and watching lots of videos related to this quest of 'going beyond the physical world'.

Why Sadhguru?

I will state at the outset that I am not associated with any particular spiritual group/institution as such and I will probably be happy to keep it that way. But of all the people that I heard, read and saw on various platforms, I was drawn towards Sadhguru for what he spoke – every single word just made so much sense. And after going through a few books of Sadhguru, I decided to take a leap of faith, straight to Sadhguru's 'energy centre'.

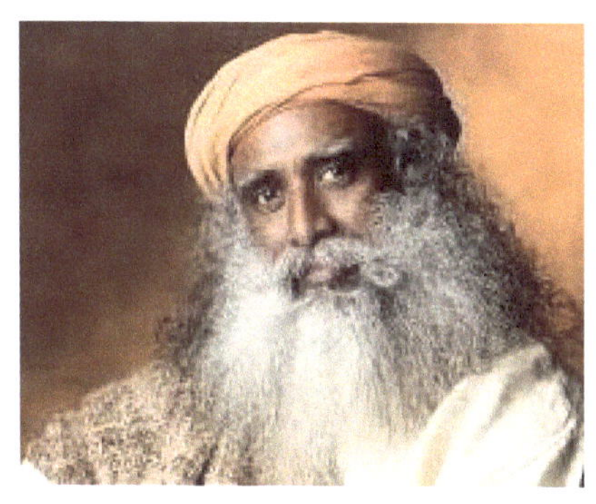

Blessings at 36000 ft

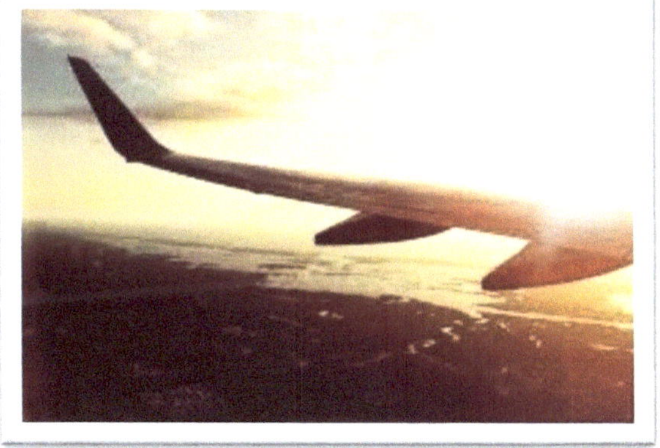

About an hour or so on my flight to Coimbatore from New Delhi, just as I started to feel a little uncomfortable, I was shifted from standard seats to the ones adjacent to the emergency exit door (with relatively better leg room) as all those seats were unoccupied and probably because I was the only one on the flight travelling alone. Then, I was the first to be served the wonderful corporate meal. Very small incidents, but since I was on a spiritual travel, I concluded, as I enjoyed my paneer wrap, that Sadhguru's magic had begun.

The first few hours

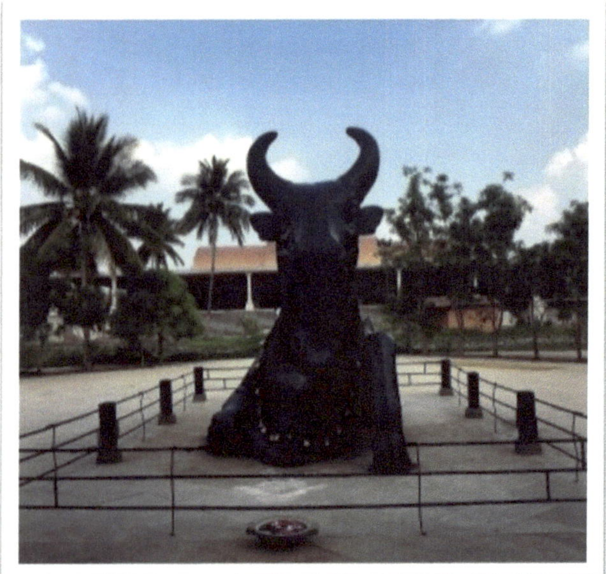
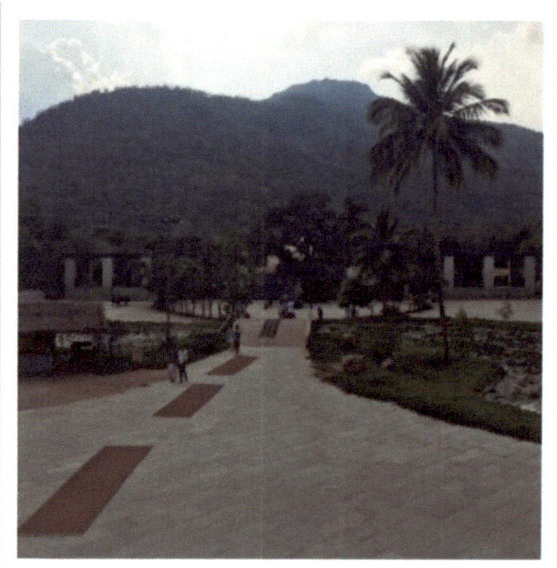

"Namaskaram Anna!" These polite words welcomed me as I entered the beautiful premises of the Isha Yoga Centre, Sadhguru Jaggi Vasudev's meditation centre at Coimbatore.
The people at the Help Desk at the main entrance were really very helpful and they quickly completed all the formalities and handed over an ID card which read 'Nadhi' (Cottage) beside my name.

On my way to my room at Nadhi cottage, I could feel the extremely soothing vibes as everyone there was so calm and smiling. After checking into my room, I immediately rushed through the map and the instruction leaflet which had information about the various activities that happen throughout the day at the centre.

Testing my luck

Soon after checking in, I was informed that it was Poornima (full moon night) that day and hence a special *pooja* (prayer) was scheduled in the evening at the Linga Bhairavi temple in the premises. I was really happy at the thought of participating in a special *pooja* that I had not even been aware of! *"Sadhguru's magic, Rahul, Sadhguru's magic"*, I whispered to myself.

And since everything seemed to be going so well that day, with utmost excitement I decided to ask the obvious question, *"Will I meet Sadhguru? Will he be there?"*

"No Anna," said the guy at the help desk very politely, *"Though Sadhguru is in the ashram today, yesterday only he met everyone at Satsang and since his diary is full of meetings/work assignments planned months ago, your meeting looks unlikely."*

I felt a bit sad. But since there were still three more days to go, I was still hopeful.

Amidst these thoughts, I headed straight to the Linga Bhairavi temple.

Actually, when you reach Isha Yoga Centre, your eyes immediately begin searching for the two popular mystic energy spots – the Linga Bhairavi temple and of course, the energy powerhouse, the Dhyanalinga, located besides the latest attraction, the 112 ft Adiyogi statue (unveiled by the honourable Prime Minister in March 2017).

One wishes to be in these spots as quickly as possible and preferably at all the three at the same time which, at least for now, is definitely beyond my capabilities (though with continued meditation, who knows)! Such was my excitement, having read so much about the mystic meditative energy around these spots.

Linga Bhairavi temple

Around 7 pm, on my way to the Linga Bhairavi temple for the special *pooja*, I passed by the Dhyanalinga. As so much was happening in my first hours at the centre, my thoughts almost froze and I was just witnessing everything, including the Dhyanlinga without any judgement or feeling, just kind of numbly, you can say.

As I reached the Linga Bhairavi temple, hundreds of shining *ghee* (clarified butter) lamps greeted me. It all looked so spectacular that I literally didn't bat an eyelid for a few seconds. As everyone calmly sat down and took their positions, *pooja* and mantra chants began and I actually felt a rush of energy just sitting there.

Linga Bhairavi, in the words of Sadhguru, is an extremely powerful feminine energy form which is very responsive for people seeking prosperity and well-being. But there is a spiritual side to Linga Bhairavi Devi as well. As I learnt from various people at the ashram, those who find it difficult to meditate when sitting in front of the Dhyanalinga, are advised to first spend some time

at the Linga Bhairavi temple as the energy there helps one to focus, and is especially beneficial during the very initial days of meditation.

Dhyanalinga

The Dhyanalinga, in the words of Sadhguru, is the largest mercury based living linga (a form or symbol) in the world which is the centre of infinite energy. In spiritual terms, in the Dhyanalinga, all aspects of life have been woven in the form of seven chakras energized to their peak and locked by Sadhguru after three years of the intense process of *prana prathistha*.

The Dhyanalinga is enshrined in a dome shaped structure of earth colour and natural stone and is in fact considered to be the best spot to meditate by the *ashram*-ites, because the energy of the Dhyanlinga is said to naturally aid you in your *dhyan* (meditation).

So much has been said and written about the unbound energy around the Dhyanalinga that for many, including myself, the Dhyanalinga is the primary reason to visit Isha Yoga Centre, at least for the first visit.

Adiyogi

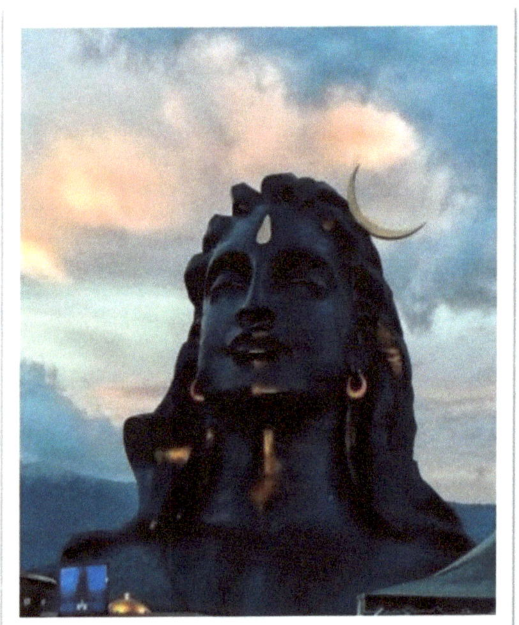

Shiva is, as we know, among the most popular and widely worshiped Indian Gods. However, after digging into the origins of yoga and meditation, including some of Sadhguru's writings, I learnt that in yogic culture, Shiva is not considered to be a God but the first yogi – the originator of yoga and the first guru (teacher) who experienced what we call 'Enlightenment' and Samadhi for the first time.

Hence, as a mark of respect and as a reminder to the world to move towards liberation through exploring the inner instead of the outer world, Sadhguru consecrated the 112 ft tall face of Adiyogi.

While I didn't find anyone meditating in front of or around Adiyogi's huge bust, there was hardly anyone visiting Isha Yoga Centre that did not spend 5-10 minutes in Adiyogi's vicinity.

The Teerthakunds – Suryakund and Chandrakund

There are two Teerthakunds or sacred water pools for purifying oneself within the Dhyanalinga complex – Suryakund for men and Chandrakund for women.

I can obviously speak of the Suryakund only that I visited, which itself looks like a divine water pool with three Shivalingas immersed in water. Ideally, men are supposed to take a dip at the Suryakund before going for meditation at the Dhyanalinga or the Linga Bhairavi temple. On the first day, I went there just for the sake of adventure but because of the powerful energy that I felt there, I could not help but take the holy bath again and again, even just before check-out.

The strong presence of the king cobra

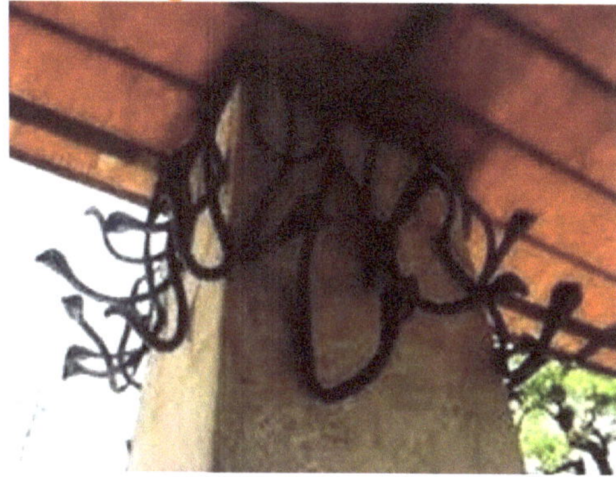

No matter where you are at Isha Yoga Centre or whatever direction you are facing, you can very strongly feel the presence of snakes (namely, king cobra) in various forms – be it representations on lamps, walls, pillars, at the Suryakund, or at the Dhyanalinga. On inquiring, I learnt that Sadhguru considers snakes, especially the king cobra to be the most sensitive animal/reptile when it comes to meditative energy. Sadhguru has also mentioned about this in his book Mystic's Musings.

Besides, since the Velliangiri Hills, where the Isha Yoga Centre is situated, are reportedly home to king cobras, the original inhabitants, in a way, Sadhguru has paid tribute to them. Luckily, I too spotted a beautiful water snake, swimming his way through the lotuses in the pond between the Nandi statue and the Suryakund.

My experience

First things first, of all the locations/energy spots at the Isha
Yoga Centre mentioned above, for me the Linga Bhairavi temple
definitely needs another mention as I spent the maximum
amount of time there and not exactly by choice. I mean there is
something really very magnetic there, something very soothing
and very, very positive, that keeps pulling you and you just
can't resist going there.

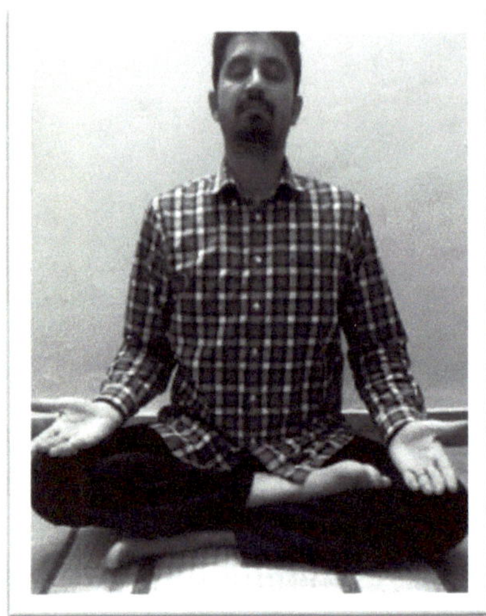

Sitting right in front of Linga Bhairavi Devi, I could actually
meditate for the longest time. More than the duration, it's the
feeling that engulfed me while meditating there. On the one
hand, I was kind of blank, absolutely calm while at the very
same time I could feel extreme joy and an unfamiliar sort of
power within. Until my last day there, I could not get enough of
meditation at the Linga Bhairavi temple. That mystic feeling is still with me.

As for the Dhyanalinga, I had read so much about it before going to Coimbatore that I had almost
made up my mind in advance that as soon as I would sit near the Dhyanalinga, I would feel
something out of the world, something really Divine. But honestly and unfortunately, I didn't feel
anything of that sort. Yes, the whole ambiance around the Dhyanalinga is very peaceful and calm
with everyone sitting in *sadhana* completely in peace and I too went to sit there again and again, at
least 8-9 times in three days, to have that out-of-the-world feeling that some people have written
about online, but I was probably not fortunate enough. In fact, as I have mentioned above, I could
feel strange energy goosebumps (giving a feeling of extreme joy) at the Linga Bhairavi temple and
even while chanting mantras at the Suryakund, but not at the Dhyanalinga.

FAQs

Finally to answer some common questions:
- **Is there really something Divine there?** Divine I don't know but yes, I felt an extreme rush
  of positive energy at some spots, especially at the Linga Bhairavi temple.

- **Will you see something beyond the physical there?** I myself didn't see or feel anything of
  that sort.

- **Will you automatically start meditating there for hours?** The whole atmosphere at the
  Isha Yoga Centre is such that meditation is all that you think of while there.

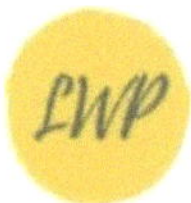

- **What exactly is taught at the Isha Yoga Centre?** There are a number of yoga programmes of varied durations happening there. Primarily, introductory programmes include Inner Engineering and Hatha Yoga while advanced programmes include Shoonya Intensive, Bhava Spandana and Samyama. Details about these programmes are available on the Isa Foundation website. I didn't attend any programme as such but one can still participate in a number of activities even without attending any programme. Among the various things that I saw and learnt there, Aumkar meditation (the correct way of uttering the sounds "Aa" , "Uu" and "Mm") and the knowledge about the various scientific facts hidden in the Mahabharta are really worth mentioning. Besides, I am now addicted to the Nirvana /Shatkam mantra and the Brahmanand Swaroopa Isha chant. They are mesmerising, really.

- **Is there any undesired commercialisation?** No, not at all. This was one concern that a few people have written about online and in fact it was also bothering me. But I am happy to write here that there is no culture of commercialisation at Isha Yoga centre. No one asks you for donation anywhere, except for a mere Rs.20 at the Suryakund which I think is legitimate for the maintenance required there.

- **Is it fine to travel with family? What about food?** There are absolutely no issues here. It's just that you go to such a place for a specific purpose, to spend maximum time meditating and hence kids can be a distraction, otherwise the stay is extremely safe and comfortable. You can book your stay at Nalanda or Nadhi cottages based on your requirement. As for the food, two meals a day are covered in your stay where you will be served simple and healthy South Indian food. For the compulsive foodies like myself, there is Peppervine Eatery within the premises which offers various delicious dishes / deserts / fresh fruit juices at a nominal price.

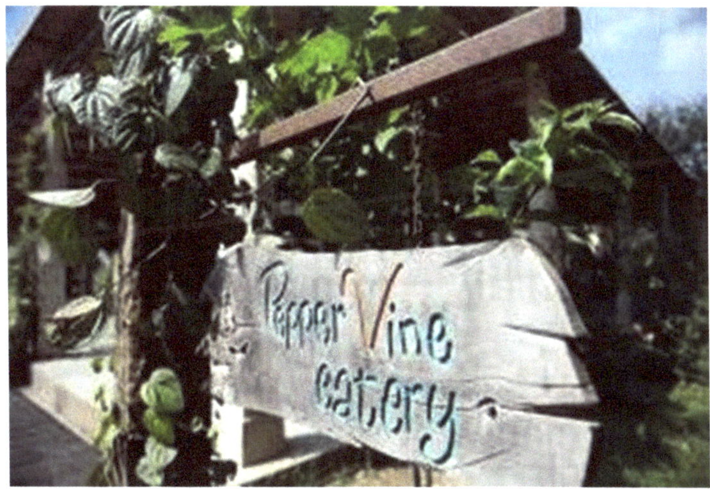

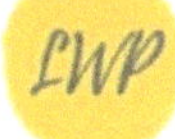

On a lighter note…

My three days were very well spent at the Isha Yoga Centre, although it would probably have been an altogether different experience had I met Sadhguru.

Nevertheless, many old questions were answered, some new ones started sprouting but a phone call at the time of check-out brought me back to square one. It was my lovely wife Nishtha. "Coimbatore's silk sarees are world famous," she said. I was supposed to understand the rest and act accordingly. Which I obviously did, to make sure that inner peace is maintained back home!

Rahul is a civil engineer by profession but an ardent traveller and a passionate blogger by choice. He practices meditation and enjoys sharing his experiences through his writing.